Sex Positions:

Understanding Sex Roles and Bedroom Bonds for Relationship Success

Lewis Finan

Table of Contents

Introduction:

In the intricate tapestry of human connection, the intimate dance between partners is a profound expression of love, desire, and vulnerability. The bedroom serves as a sacred space where bonds are forged, pleasures are explored, and communication transcends words. "Sex Positions: Understanding Sex Roles and Bedroom Bonds for Relationship Success" is an exploration into the art and science of physical intimacy, aimed at fostering deeper connections and promoting relationship success.

This book delves beyond the surface of traditional discussions on sex, seeking to unravel the complexities of sexual roles and dynamics within the context of a loving relationship. It is a guide that goes beyond the physical aspects of sex, delving into the emotional, psychological, and relational dimensions that contribute to a fulfilling and harmonious partnership.

Sexual positions are not merely physical configurations; they are expressions of communication, trust, and vulnerability. Each position tells a story, conveys an emotion, and serves as a vessel for mutual understanding. By unraveling the intricacies of these positions, we can uncover the subtle nuances that define the unique language of intimacy shared by two individuals.

As we embark on this journey, we will explore how sex roles have evolved through time, reflecting societal changes and challenging traditional norms. The book navigates through the diverse landscape of sexual preferences, desires, and fantasies, emphasizing the importance of open communication and consent in the pursuit of mutual pleasure and satisfaction.

"Sex Positions" is not a manual dictating rigid rules; instead, it encourages a dynamic and personalized approach to physical connection. It provides a roadmap for couples to explore their desires, experiment with different positions, and adapt them to suit their unique preferences. The goal is not only to enhance pleasure but to deepen emotional bonds, fostering a sense of intimacy that transcends the physical act.

Throughout these pages, we will draw upon insights from experts, personal narratives, and research to illuminate the multifaceted nature of human sexuality. We will challenge preconceived notions, celebrate diversity, and offer guidance for navigating the complexities of intimacy within the framework of a committed relationship.

Join us on this exploration of passion, connection, and self-discovery. "Sex Positions" is an invitation to cultivate a deeper understanding of yourself and your partner, fostering a relationship that stands the test of time and flourishes in both and out of the bedroom.

Opening Remarks

Welcome to a journey that transcends the boundaries of physical intimacy and ventures into the intricate realm of human relationships. As we embark on the pages of "Sex Positions: Understanding Sex Roles and Bedroom Bonds for Relationship Success," we open the door to a conversation that goes beyond the surface, delving into the complexities of love, desire, and the unique language spoken between partners.

In the sanctuary of the bedroom, we discover a canvas where emotions are painted, trust is sculpted, and communication becomes an art form. This book is not merely a guide to sexual positions; it is an exploration of the nuanced dance that occurs when two souls intertwine in a shared pursuit of connection and pleasure.

Through these pages, we invite you to challenge preconceived notions, embrace diversity, and navigate the evolving landscape of sexual roles. Our goal is to provide a roadmap for couples to embark on a journey of self-discovery, mutual understanding, and a flourishing connection that extends far beyond the confines of physical intimacy.

In the spirit of openness, respect, and celebration of the unique dynamics that define each relationship, let us delve into the heart of "Sex Positions." May this exploration ignite conversations, foster understanding, and ultimately contribute to the success and fulfillment of your relationships.

With anticipation and excitement for the revelations that lie ahead, welcome to a transformative exploration of love and connection.

Let the journey begin.

Purpose of the Book

The purpose of "Sex Positions: Understanding Sex Roles and Bedroom Bonds for Relationship Success" is multifaceted and deeply rooted in the aspiration to enhance the quality and depth of intimate connections between partners. This book aims to serve as a guide, an inspiration, and a source of knowledge, addressing several key purposes:

Fostering Communication and Understanding:

The book seeks to promote open and honest communication between partners about their desires, preferences, and boundaries. By exploring various sex positions, it encourages couples to engage in conversations that go beyond the physical, deepening their understanding of each other's needs and fostering emotional intimacy.

Promoting Relationship Success:

Recognizing that a strong physical connection is often a reflection of a healthy relationship, the book provides insights and guidance to contribute to overall relationship success. It emphasizes the interconnectedness of emotional, psychological, and physical aspects of intimacy, striving to create a harmonious balance that enhances the well-being of both partners.

Celebrating Diversity and Individuality:

In acknowledging the uniqueness of every relationship, the book celebrates diversity in sexual preferences and roles. It encourages readers to embrace their individuality and that of their partners, fostering an environment where personal exploration is not only accepted but celebrated as a vital component of a thriving relationship.

Empowering Couples through Knowledge:

By combining expert insights, research findings, and real-life narratives, the book empowers couples with knowledge. It equips them with a comprehensive understanding of the multifaceted nature of human sexuality, encouraging informed decision-making, and inspiring a sense of confidence in exploring and expressing their desires.

Encouraging Sensual Creativity and Playfulness:

"Sex Positions" aims to inject a sense of playfulness and creativity into intimate relationships. By presenting a variety of positions as a palette for exploration, the book encourages couples to experiment, discover, and create a shared language of pleasure that evolves over time.

Addressing Changing Societal Norms:

Recognizing the evolving nature of societal norms and expectations, the book navigates through the historical context of sex roles. It encourages readers to critically examine and challenge traditional perspectives, fostering an inclusive and progressive approach to intimate relationships.

In essence, the purpose of this book is to guide couples on a transformative journey—one that goes beyond the physical act of sex and into the realms of mutual understanding, appreciation, and enduring connection. It is a resource designed to empower individuals and couples alike to navigate the complexities of intimacy with wisdom, compassion, and a profound appreciation for the beauty of human connection.

Chapter 1: Foundations of Intimacy

In the vast landscape of human connection, intimacy serves as the bedrock upon which profound relationships are built. This chapter invites you to embark on a journey into the fundamental elements that underpin a strong and fulfilling intimate connection between partners.

Defining Intimacy:

To lay the groundwork, we delve into the multifaceted concept of intimacy. What does it mean to be truly intimate with another person? From emotional vulnerability to shared secrets, we explore the various dimensions that contribute to the rich tapestry of intimacy.

The Emotional Landscape:

Intimacy extends far beyond the physical realm, encompassing a rich emotional landscape. This section explores the power of emotional connection, the role of trust, and the significance of understanding and responding to each other's needs.

Communication as the Cornerstone:

Effective communication is the cornerstone of any strong relationship. Here, we delve into the importance of open and honest dialogue, providing practical tips and tools to enhance communication skills, and ensuring that partners feel heard and understood.

The Intersection of Trust and Vulnerability:

Trust and vulnerability are inseparable companions on the journey to intimacy. We navigate the delicate balance between opening oneself up to another and fostering an environment of trust, examining how these elements intertwine to create a foundation for deep connection.

Cultural and Societal Influences:

Understanding the impact of cultural and societal norms on intimacy is crucial. This section examines how external influences shape our perceptions of intimacy, challenging preconceived notions and encouraging a nuanced approach to building connections within diverse contexts.

The Evolution of Intimacy:

As we journey through history, we explore how societal changes have influenced the dynamics of intimacy. From traditional roles to contemporary expectations, this section provides insight into the evolving nature of intimate relationships and the adaptability required for enduring connections.

The Role of Sex in Intimacy:

While sex is just one facet of intimacy, it holds a unique place in the relational landscape. We begin to explore the interplay between emotional connection and physical expression, setting the stage for a deeper examination in subsequent chapters.

Exercises for Connection:

To bring the theoretical into the practical, this chapter concludes with exercises designed to enhance intimacy. From communication exercises to activities fostering vulnerability, these practical tools provide a hands-on approach to strengthening the foundations of your relationship.

As we navigate the foundations of intimacy, let this chapter serve as a compass, guiding you toward a deeper understanding of the emotional, psychological, and cultural elements that contribute to the profound tapestry of connection between you and your partner. In the chapters that follow, we will continue to unravel the intricate threads that weave together to create lasting and meaningful relationships.

1.1 Exploring Emotional Connection

In the intricate dance of human connection, the heartbeat of intimacy resonates in the emotional bonds that bind individuals together. The exploration of emotional connection is a profound journey into the core of relationships, transcending physicality to delve into the depths of vulnerability, understanding, and shared experiences. This chapter peels back the layers of emotional intimacy, examining its significance, intricacies, and the ways in which it shapes the foundation of lasting and meaningful connections.

1. *Understanding Emotional Connection:*

At the heart of emotional connection lies the ability to understand and be understood on a profound level. It surpasses mere verbal communication, extending into the realms of empathy, attunement, and the recognition of one another's innermost thoughts and feelings. Emotional connection is the invisible thread that weaves together the fabric of a relationship, creating a sense of safety and acceptance.

2. *The Power of Vulnerability:*

Vulnerability is the currency of emotional connection. It is the courageous act of revealing one's authentic self, fears, and insecurities to another. In this section, we explore the transformative power of vulnerability, acknowledging that it is through openness and shared vulnerability that a deep emotional connection flourishes.

3. *The Role of Trust in Emotional Intimacy:*

Trust is the bedrock upon which emotional connection is built. This section dissects the components of trust – reliability, consistency, and integrity – emphasizing its pivotal role in fostering an environment where individuals feel secure enough to share their innermost thoughts and feelings without fear of judgment or betrayal.

4. Emotional Communication:

While communication is a broad concept, this section hones in on the nuances of emotional communication. It explores the language of emotions, the importance of active listening, and the role of non-verbal cues in conveying feelings. Effective emotional communication lays the groundwork for a deeper understanding of one another's emotional worlds.

5. Emotional Intelligence:

Emotional intelligence, the ability to perceive, understand, and manage one's own emotions and the emotions of others, is a key factor in building and sustaining emotional connection. This section explores the components of emotional intelligence and how developing this skill set can enhance the quality of emotional bonds within a relationship.

6. Navigating Emotional Differences:

Individuals bring unique emotional landscapes to a relationship, shaped by personal experiences, upbringing, and temperament. Navigating these differences requires a blend of empathy and acceptance. This section provides insights into understanding and appreciating the diversity of emotional expressions within a partnership.

7. *The Impact of Past Experiences:*

Emotional connection is often influenced by past experiences, both positive and negative. This section delves into the ways in which past relationships, family dynamics, and personal history can shape an individual's ability to connect emotionally and provides guidance on navigating the impact of these experiences on current relationships.

8. *Rituals of Connection:*

Building and maintaining emotional connection requires intentional efforts. Rituals of connection, whether they be daily check-ins, shared activities, or expressions of affection, play a crucial role in nurturing the emotional bond between partners. This section explores the significance of these rituals and offers suggestions for incorporating them into daily life.

9. *Nurturing Emotional Intimacy:*

As we conclude our exploration, the focus turns to practical strategies for nurturing emotional intimacy. From cultivating gratitude to fostering a culture of appreciation, this section provides actionable steps for individuals and couples to strengthen the emotional connection that forms the heart of their relationship.

In unraveling the layers of emotional connection, we uncover the essence of what it means to truly know and be known by another. Emotional intimacy is not a static state but a dynamic journey of continuous exploration, understanding, and growth. As we navigate the intricate terrain of emotions within the context of relationships, may this exploration inspire a deeper commitment to fostering emotional connections that stand the test of time.

1.2 Communication in the Bedroom

In the private realm of the bedroom, where desires intertwine and passions unfold, effective communication serves as the cornerstone for a fulfilling and harmonious sexual connection. This chapter delves into the intricate dynamics of communication within the intimate space, exploring how verbal and non-verbal expressions can bridge the gap between partners, enhance mutual understanding, and elevate the overall experience of intimacy.

1. Verbal Communication: The Language of Desires

Communication in the bedroom begins with the spoken word. This section emphasizes the importance of clear and open verbal communication about desires, boundaries, and preferences. It explores ways in which partners can express their needs with honesty and sensitivity, fostering an environment where both voices are heard and respected.

2. Active Listening: The Art of Presence

As crucial as expressing one's desires is the art of active listening. Understanding and responding to verbal cues, as well as tuning in to non-verbal signals, deepens the connection between partners. This section provides insights into the transformative power of being fully present, attentive, and responsive to each other's verbal expressions.

3. Non-Verbal Communication: The Silent Symphony

Sometimes, the most profound communication occurs without words. This section delves into the world of non-verbal cues – the subtle touches, glances, and body language that convey a wealth of emotions and desires. It explores the significance of non-verbal communication in creating an intimate connection that goes beyond the limitations of language.

4. Consent and Communication: Building Trust

Consent is a fundamental aspect of any healthy sexual relationship. This section explores the vital role communication plays in obtaining and giving consent. It emphasizes the ongoing nature of consent, the need for clear communication about boundaries, and the creation of a trusting environment where both partners feel secure and respected.

5. Expressing Fantasies and Desires: Mutual Exploration

The bedroom is a canvas for exploration and shared fantasies. This section encourages partners to communicate openly about their desires and fantasies, fostering an atmosphere of mutual exploration and acceptance. It provides guidance on initiating conversations about fantasies, creating a space where both partners feel comfortable expressing their deepest desires.

6. Communication During Intimacy: The Dance of Connection

Communication doesn't cease when physical intimacy begins; it evolves into a non-verbal dance of connection. This section explores the ways in which partners can communicate during moments of intimacy, using subtle cues and feedback to enhance the shared experience. It emphasizes the importance of attunement and responsiveness in deepening the connection between partners.

7. Addressing Challenges: Navigating Difficult Conversations

No relationship is without its challenges. This section provides guidance on navigating difficult conversations in the bedroom, whether it be addressing performance concerns, exploring new territories, or discussing changes in desire. Effective communication becomes a tool for understanding, empathy, and finding solutions that strengthen the bond between partners.

8. Building a Language of Intimacy: Consistency and Adaptability

Consistency in communication builds a stable foundation, while adaptability ensures that the language of intimacy remains dynamic. This section explores the balance between consistency and adaptability, encouraging partners to evolve their communication styles as the relationship grows and changes.

9. Exercises for Enhanced Communication: Practical Applications

To translate theory into practice, this chapter concludes with practical exercises aimed at enhancing communication in the bedroom. From guided conversations to shared activities, these exercises provide tangible tools for partners to deepen their connection and strengthen the communicative bonds within their intimate relationship.

In the realm of sexual intimacy, effective communication is the linchpin that transforms physical acts into shared expressions of love, desire, and connection. As we navigate the intricacies of communication in the bedroom, may this exploration inspire partners to build bridges of understanding, fostering a sexual connection that is not only pleasurable but also deeply fulfilling and enriching.

Chapter 2: The Dynamics of Desire

Desire, the magnetic force that draws individuals together, weaves a complex tapestry within the intimate fabric of relationships. This chapter unravels the intricate dynamics of desire, exploring its various dimensions, sources, and the ways in which it shapes the ebb and flow of intimacy between partners.

1. Defining Desire: The Essence of Connection

At the heart of desire lies an intrinsic longing for connection. This section delves into the multifaceted nature of desire, examining its emotional, psychological, and physical components. By understanding desire as a dynamic force, partners can embark on a journey to explore and nurture the diverse facets of their shared longing.

2. Sources of Desire: Unraveling the Threads

Desire is a product of numerous influences, both internal and external. This section explores the sources of desire, from individual fantasies to societal expectations. By unraveling these threads, partners can gain insight into the diverse factors that shape their desires and contribute to a richer understanding of each other's unique longings.

3. The Interplay of Emotional and Physical Desire

Emotional and physical desires dance in a delicate interplay, each influencing the other. This section examines how emotional intimacy can fuel physical desire and vice versa. By recognizing the symbiotic relationship between these two dimensions, partners can cultivate a more holistic approach to desire within their relationship.

4. Understanding Variability: Peaks and Valleys of Desire

Desire is not a static force; it ebbs and flows over time. This section explores the natural variability of desire within relationships, acknowledging that fluctuations are a normal part of the human experience. By understanding the rhythms of desire, partners can navigate its peaks and valleys with compassion and open communication.

5. Communicating Desires: The Art of Vulnerability

Expressing desires requires a delicate balance of vulnerability and openness. This section delves into the art of communicating desires, encouraging partners to share their fantasies, preferences, and needs with authenticity. Effective communication becomes a bridge that connects the intricate landscape of desires, fostering a deeper connection.

6. Resolving Desire Discrepancies: Bridging the Gap

Desire discrepancies are common within relationships, posing both challenges and opportunities for growth. This section provides guidance on navigating differences in desire, fostering understanding, and finding collaborative solutions. By viewing desire as a shared exploration, partners can transform challenges into opportunities for mutual satisfaction.

7. *Embracing Diversity: Beyond Societal Norms*

Societal norms often shape our perceptions of desire, imposing expectations that may not align with individual or relational realities. This section encourages partners to embrace the diversity of desires within their relationship, challenging societal norms and fostering an inclusive environment where both partners feel validated and accepted.

8. *Eroticism and Intimacy: Navigating the Connection*

Eroticism, the poetic dance of sensuality and desire, plays a pivotal role in intimate relationships. This section explores the connection between eroticism and intimacy, emphasizing the importance of cultivating a space where partners can explore their sensual desires freely and without judgment.

9. *Cultivating a Culture of Desire: Practical Strategies*

To bring the exploration of desire into practical application, this chapter concludes with actionable strategies for cultivating a culture of desire within a relationship. From creating shared fantasies to introducing variety, these strategies provide partners with tools to invigorate and sustain the dynamics of desire over time.

In unraveling the complexities of desire, this chapter invites partners to embark on a shared journey of exploration, understanding, and celebration. By navigating the intricate dance of desire, couples can foster a connection that not only withstands the test of time but flourishes in the ever-evolving landscape of their intimate relationship.

2.1 Unveiling Personal Preferences

In the realm of intimate relationships, the exploration of personal preferences is an intimate journey that involves vulnerability, communication, and a shared commitment to mutual satisfaction. This chapter delves into the intricate process of unveiling personal preferences, encouraging partners to navigate this landscape with sensitivity, curiosity, and a willingness to embrace the uniqueness of each other's desires.

1. Acknowledging Individual Desires: The Tapestry of Uniqueness

Every individual carries a unique tapestry of desires, shaped by personal experiences, fantasies, and emotional landscapes. This section emphasizes the importance of acknowledging and embracing individual desires as an essential aspect of self-discovery within the context of a relationship. By recognizing and valuing these differences, partners lay the foundation for a more intimate and understanding connection.

2. Creating a Safe Space: Fostering Open Communication

Unveiling personal preferences requires a safe and judgment-free space for open communication. This section explores the dynamics of creating an environment where partners feel comfortable expressing their desires without fear of criticism or rejection. Effective communication becomes the key to understanding, acceptance, and the mutual exploration of intimate preferences.

3. The Language of Desires: Verbal Expression

Verbal expression is a powerful tool in the unveiling of personal preferences. This section delves into the art of using language to communicate desires, fantasies, and boundaries. Partners are encouraged to find their unique verbal language, fostering a deeper understanding of each other's wants and needs.

4. Non-Verbal Cues: The Silent Language of Intimacy

While words convey desires, non-verbal cues play an equally vital role in unveiling personal preferences. This section explores the silent language of intimacy, examining the significance of body language, gestures, and subtle cues in expressing and interpreting desires. Partners are invited to attune themselves to these non-verbal expressions, enriching their connection on a profound level.

5. Encouraging Exploration: Mutual Curiosity and Respect

The journey of unveiling personal preferences is a shared exploration. This section emphasizes the importance of mutual curiosity and respect in discovering and understanding each other's desires. By approaching this exploration with an open mind and a sense of adventure, partners can foster a dynamic and evolving intimacy that continually enriches their connection.

6. Respecting Boundaries: Balancing Exploration and Comfort

As partners navigate the landscape of personal preferences, it's crucial to respect boundaries. This section explores the delicate balance between exploration and comfort, encouraging open communication about limits and ensuring that both partners feel secure and respected in their intimate interactions.

7. Celebrating Diversity: Embracing the Spectrum of Desires

Each individual brings a unique spectrum of desires to the relationship. This section invites partners to celebrate this diversity, recognizing that it adds depth and richness to the shared experience of intimacy. By embracing the spectrum of desires, couples can cultivate an environment that nurtures both individuality and togetherness.

8. *Addressing Discrepancies: Finding Common Ground*

Desire discrepancies are a natural part of intimate relationships. This section provides insights into addressing disparities in preferences, fostering understanding, and finding common ground. Partners are encouraged to view these differences as opportunities for negotiation, compromise, and the evolution of a shared language of intimacy.

9. *Mutual Growth: Evolving Together*

Unveiling personal preferences is not a static process but an ongoing journey of mutual growth. This section explores the concept of evolving together, encouraging partners to be receptive to changing desires, interests, and needs. The willingness to adapt and grow ensures that the intimate connection remains vibrant and fulfilling over time.

In the delicate dance of unveiling personal preferences, partners embark on a journey of self-discovery and shared exploration. By navigating this landscape with sensitivity, open communication, and a commitment to understanding, couples can forge a deeper connection that transcends the boundaries of the known and opens doors to new dimensions of intimacy.

2.2 Understanding Libido

Libido, often described as the spark that ignites passion, is a nuanced aspect of human sexuality that ebbs and flows within the currents of life. This exploration delves into the multifaceted nature of libido, offering insights into its sources, variations, and the ways in which partners can navigate its fluctuations in the pursuit of a harmonious and fulfilling sexual connection.

1. Defining Libido: The Essence of Sexual Vitality

Libido, at its core, is the energy that propels individuals toward sexual expression. This section provides a foundational understanding of libido as a dynamic force that encompasses both physical and psychological components. By recognizing libido as a vital aspect of overall well-being, partners can approach its exploration with sensitivity and awareness.

2. The Factors Influencing Libido: A Complex Tapestry

Numerous factors weave into the intricate tapestry of libido. This section explores the diverse influences, including hormonal fluctuations, stress, health, relationship dynamics, and life events. Understanding these factors is essential for partners seeking to navigate the complexities of libido fluctuations and foster a supportive environment for each other's sexual vitality.

3. Individual Variances: Recognizing Diverse Sexual Rhythms

Individuals possess unique sexual rhythms, contributing to variations in libido levels. This section encourages partners to appreciate and respect these variances, recognizing that differences in libido are a natural aspect of human sexuality. By acknowledging and understanding each other's unique rhythms, couples can cultivate a compassionate and accepting approach to sexual desire.

4. Emotional Intimacy and Libido: The Interplay

The quality of emotional intimacy within a relationship significantly influences libido. This section explores the intricate interplay between emotional connection and sexual desire, highlighting the importance of cultivating a nurturing emotional environment. Partners are encouraged to foster communication, trust, and vulnerability as foundational elements that support a healthy libido.

5. Stress and Libido: Navigating Life's Pressures

Stress, a ubiquitous element of modern life, can impact libido in profound ways. This section delves into the relationship between stress and sexual desire, offering strategies for partners to navigate life's pressures collaboratively. By creating a supportive atmosphere during stressful times, couples can mitigate the effects of stress on libido and strengthen their connection.

6. Health and Lifestyle: The Impact on Sexual Vitality

Physical health and lifestyle choices play a crucial role in libido. This section explores the ways in which factors such as exercise, nutrition, and overall well-being contribute to sexual vitality. Partners are encouraged to embark on a shared journey of prioritizing health, recognizing its positive effects on both individual and mutual libido.

7. Communication about Libido: Fostering Understanding

Open communication is paramount when navigating the ebbs and flows of libido. This section provides guidance on initiating conversations about sexual desire, and encouraging partners to express their needs, concerns, and desires with empathy and honesty. Effective communication becomes a bridge that connects partners and enhances their ability to navigate the intricate landscape of libido.

8. Libido Discrepancies: Navigating Challenges Together

Libido discrepancies are a common aspect of intimate relationships. This section offers insights into addressing differences in sexual desire, emphasizing the importance of empathy, patience, and collaborative problem-solving. Partners are encouraged to view libido challenges as opportunities for growth, understanding, and the evolution of a resilient sexual connection.

9. Cultivating a Libido-Friendly Relationship: Practical Strategies

To bring theoretical understanding into practical application, this chapter concludes with actionable strategies for cultivating a libido-friendly relationship. From creating a sensual environment to prioritizing intimate moments, these strategies provide partners with tangible tools to enhance sexual vitality and foster a connection that transcends the fluctuations of libido.

In unraveling the nuances of libido, partners embark on a journey of mutual understanding, empathy, and shared exploration. By navigating the ebb and flow of sexual desire with compassion and awareness, couples can cultivate a vibrant and enduring sexual connection that aligns with the ever-changing rhythms of life and love.

Chapter 3: Sex Roles and Relationship Dynamics

Within the intricate dance of intimate partnerships, the roles individuals assume play a significant role in shaping the dynamics of a relationship. This chapter delves into the complex interplay of sex roles—defined by societal expectations—and the evolving dynamics that emerge within the private spaces of love and connection.

1. Unpacking Sex Roles: Societal Expectations and Influences

This section initiates the exploration by unraveling the concept of sex roles, delving into the societal expectations and influences that shape traditional gender roles. Understanding the historical context and prevailing norms provides a foundation for a nuanced discussion on the impact of these roles on contemporary relationships.

2. Evolving Dynamics: The Shifting Landscape of Relationships

As societal norms transform, so do the dynamics within relationships. This section examines the evolving landscape of partnerships, exploring how modern relationships challenge and redefine traditional sex roles. Partners are encouraged to reflect on their roles and expectations, fostering a dynamic and adaptable approach to shared responsibilities.

3. Communication Styles: Bridging the Gap

Sex roles often influence communication styles within relationships. This section navigates the nuances of how gendered expectations may shape the ways in which partners express themselves, fostering an understanding of the potential impact on effective communication. Strategies for bridging communication gaps and promoting open dialogue are explored.

4. Balancing Responsibilities: Shared Roles and Collaborative Partnerships

Achieving balance in shared responsibilities is a key theme in this section. Partnerships thrive when roles are shared, and responsibilities are distributed equitably. The chapter explores the benefits of collaborative decision-making, emphasizing the importance of flexibility and adaptability in navigating the ever-changing landscape of modern relationships.

5. Intimacy and Vulnerability: Breaking Down Stereotypes

Traditional sex roles can influence perceptions of intimacy and vulnerability. This section challenges stereotypes that may hinder emotional expression, encouraging partners to embrace vulnerability as a strength. By dismantling preconceived notions, couples can create an environment that fosters deep emotional connections.

6. *Power Dynamics: Navigating Equality*

Power dynamics within relationships are a reflection of sex roles and societal expectations. This section examines the quest for equality in partnerships, encouraging partners to recognize and address imbalances. Strategies for fostering a sense of equality in decision-making, support, and influence are explored.

7. *Sexual Expression: Embracing Individual Desires*

Sex roles can impact sexual expression, shaping expectations around desire and initiation. This section encourages partners to explore and express their individual desires, free from restrictive gender norms. By embracing the diversity of sexual expression, couples can create a space where both partners feel empowered to communicate their needs.

8. *Parenting Roles: Navigating Parenthood as Partners*

The dynamics of sex roles often become pronounced in the realm of parenting. This section explores how traditional expectations may influence parenting roles and offers guidance on fostering collaborative and supportive approaches to co-parenting. Strategies for navigating challenges and creating a unified front are discussed.

9. *Redefining Success: Shared Goals and Mutual Growth*

Success within a relationship is redefined when partners collaboratively set and pursue shared goals. This section explores the importance of aligning aspirations, celebrating individual achievements, and fostering an environment where both partners can experience personal and mutual growth.

In navigating the terrain of sex roles and relationship dynamics, this chapter invites partners to critically examine societal expectations, challenge traditional norms, and foster a relationship environment that is adaptable, communicative, and supportive. By embracing evolving roles and mutual respect, couples can co-create a dynamic partnership that thrives in the face of societal shifts and individual growth.

3.1 Traditional vs. Modern Perspectives

As relationships evolve in the ever-changing tapestry of society, contrasting perspectives—traditional and modern—shape the dynamics of intimate partnerships. This exploration delves into the nuances of these perspectives, examining how societal shifts influence the expectations, roles, and values within relationships.

1. *Traditional Perspectives: Foundations of the Past*

Traditional perspectives on relationships are deeply rooted in historical norms and societal structures. This section delves into the historical context that has shaped conventional expectations, roles, and power dynamics within intimate partnerships. Understanding the foundation of traditional perspectives provides insight into the origins of long-standing norms.

2. Modern Perspectives: Embracing Change and Diversity

The modern era witnessed a transformative shift in societal norms, challenging and reshaping traditional perspectives. This section explores the contemporary landscape of relationships, emphasizing the embrace of diversity, equality, and fluid roles. Modern perspectives celebrate individuality and encourage couples to forge partnerships based on mutual respect and shared values.

3. Relationship Structures: From Conventional to Varied Forms

Traditional perspectives often dictate conventional relationship structures, emphasizing monogamy and specific gender roles. In contrast, modern perspectives open the door to diverse relationship forms, including non-traditional partnerships, polyamory, and a spectrum of gender expressions. This section examines the evolving landscape, encouraging couples to explore structures that resonate with their values and desires.

4. Gender Roles: Breaking Free from Stereotypes

Traditional perspectives often prescribe rigid gender roles, influencing expectations about behavior, responsibilities, and expressions of intimacy. The modern view challenges these stereotypes, promoting equality and fluidity in gender roles. Partners are encouraged to navigate the space between tradition and modernity, fostering relationships that celebrate the uniqueness of each individual.

5. Communication Styles: From Reserved to Open Dialogues

Traditional communication styles may prioritize discretion and avoidance of certain topics. In the modern era, an emphasis is placed on open and honest communication. This section explores the evolution of communication styles, advocating for partners to cultivate an environment where dialogue is encouraged, vulnerabilities are shared, and understanding deepens.

6. Decision-Making Dynamics: Collaborative vs. Authoritative Approaches

Traditional relationships may lean towards authoritative decision-making, influenced by defined roles. Modern relationships, however, often embrace collaborative decision-making, where partners share responsibilities and contribute equally to choices. This section navigates the shift in decision-making dynamics, highlighting the benefits of mutual collaboration and compromise.

7. Work-Life Balance: Integrating Professional and Personal Lives

Traditional perspectives often compartmentalize work and personal life, while modern approaches seek a more integrated balance. This section explores the changing attitudes toward career, family, and personal pursuits, encouraging couples to co-create a balance that aligns with their individual and shared aspirations.

8. Intimacy and Sexuality: Liberation from Taboos

Traditional perspectives may impose taboos and expectations on intimacy and sexuality. Modern perspectives celebrate sexual liberation, advocating for open communication, consent, and the exploration of diverse expressions of desire. Partners are invited to navigate this evolution, fostering an environment where intimacy is consensual, respectful, and pleasurable for both individuals.

9. Parenthood and Family Structures: Redefining Roles

Traditional perspectives often dictate rigid roles in parenthood and family structures. Modern approaches challenge these norms, promoting shared responsibilities, flexible roles, and diverse family compositions. This section explores the redefinition of roles within the family unit, emphasizing the importance of mutual support and adaptability.

In navigating the intricate interplay between traditional and modern perspectives, couples are invited to reflect on their values, communicate openly, and co-create a relationship that aligns with the evolving landscape of societal expectations. By embracing diversity, equality, and shared growth, partners can forge a resilient connection that stands the test of time and adapts to the changing currents of contemporary life.

3.2 Navigating Gender Roles

In the intricate dance of intimate partnerships, the exploration of gender roles unfolds as a dynamic and evolving journey. This chapter delves into the complexities of navigating gender roles, encouraging couples to embrace diversity, challenge stereotypes, and foster relationships built on equality and mutual respect.

1. Understanding Gender Roles: Historical Context and Evolution

To navigate gender roles effectively, an exploration of their historical context is paramount. This section delves into the evolution of traditional gender roles, acknowledging how societal expectations have shaped perceptions of masculinity and femininity. Understanding this foundation provides a basis for reexamining and reshaping contemporary perspectives.

2. Embracing Gender Diversity: Beyond Binary Definitions

Modern relationships transcend binary definitions of gender. This section explores the expanding spectrum of gender identities and expressions, inviting partners to embrace diversity. By acknowledging and celebrating the richness of gender diversity, couples create a foundation for inclusivity within their relationship.

3. Breaking Stereotypes: Challenging Conventional Expectations

Stereotypes surrounding gender roles can limit the potential for authentic self-expression. This section encourages partners to challenge and break free from conventional expectations, fostering an environment where each individual is empowered to express their unique qualities and strengths regardless of societal norms.

4. Equality in Responsibilities: Collaborative Partnerships

Achieving equality in responsibilities is a key theme in this chapter. Partnerships thrive when both individuals actively contribute to shared responsibilities, unburdened by predefined gender roles. The section explores the benefits of collaborative decision-making, recognizing the strengths each partner brings to the relationship.

5. Communication Styles: Bridging the Gender Gap

Gender roles often influence communication styles within relationships. This section navigates the nuances of how societal expectations may shape the ways in which partners express themselves. By fostering open and empathetic communication, couples bridge the gender gap and create a space for genuine understanding.

6. *Intimacy and Emotional Expression: Beyond Traditional Boundaries*

Traditional gender roles may dictate specific modes of emotional expression and intimacy. This section explores how partners can transcend these boundaries, fostering an environment where emotional vulnerability and intimacy are celebrated in diverse ways. Couples are encouraged to create a space where both partners feel free to express their emotions authentically.

7. *Career and Ambitions: Supporting Individual Aspirations*

Gender roles can influence expectations surrounding careers and ambitions. This section advocates for supporting each other's individual aspirations, irrespective of gender. Partners are encouraged to foster an environment where professional pursuits align with personal goals, unencumbered by traditional stereotypes.

8. *Decision-Making Dynamics: Shared Leadership and Empowerment*

The chapter examines the evolution of decision-making dynamics within relationships. Modern partnerships embrace shared leadership, empowering both individuals to actively contribute to choices that shape their lives. By fostering an environment of mutual empowerment, couples navigate decisions collaboratively, drawing strength from the diversity of their perspectives.

9. Parenting Roles: Nurturing Beyond Traditional Norms

Parenting roles are often influenced by traditional gender expectations. This section explores how couples can redefine parenting roles, encouraging shared responsibilities and nurturing styles. By challenging stereotypes, partners create an environment where both parents actively participate in the growth and well-being of their children.

In navigating gender roles, couples embark on a journey of self-discovery, mutual understanding, and shared growth. By embracing diversity, challenging stereotypes, and fostering equality, partners co-create a relationship that celebrates the richness of individual identity and allows for the evolution of gender roles in sync with the ever-changing landscape of contemporary relationships.

Chapter 4: Exploring Sex Positions

Within the sacred space of intimate connection, the exploration of sex positions unfolds as a deeply personal and sensual journey. This chapter delves into the art of exploring sex positions, inviting couples to embark on a voyage that not only enhances physical pleasure but also fosters a profound intimacy within their relationship.

1. The Language of Bodies: Beyond the Physical Act

Sex positions transcend the physical act itself; they are a language through which partners communicate desire, vulnerability, and passion. This section explores the emotional and psychological dimensions of sex positions, emphasizing the role they play in creating a shared narrative of intimacy.

2. Connection and Trust: Foundations of Pleasure

Before delving into specific positions, it's essential to establish the foundations of connection and trust. This section emphasizes the importance of open communication, consent, and a deep emotional bond as the groundwork for a fulfilling exploration of sex positions.

3. Variety as the Spice of Intimacy: Beyond Routine

Variety is the spice that invigorates intimate relationships. This section encourages couples to move beyond routine, exploring different sex positions to discover what resonates with their desires and brings novelty to their shared experiences.

4. Finding Comfort: Balancing Exploration and Ease

While variety is encouraged, finding comfort in exploration is equally vital. This section provides insights into balancing the excitement of trying new positions with the importance of ensuring physical comfort and emotional well-being for both partners.

5. Enhancing Pleasure: The Art of Mutual Satisfaction

Sex positions are a canvas for enhancing pleasure and mutual satisfaction. This section explores the intricacies of positions that cater to the diverse needs and desires of both partners, fostering an environment where pleasure is a shared and reciprocal experience.

6. Intimacy Beyond Penetrative Sex: Expanding the Repertoire

Intimacy extends beyond penetrative sex, and this section delves into the exploration of non-penetrative positions. From sensual massages to intimate embraces, couples are encouraged to broaden their repertoire, fostering a holistic approach to physical connection.

7. Communication During Intimacy: Tuning into Non-Verbal Cues

Non-verbal communication plays a significant role during intimate moments. This section explores how partners can tune into each other's non-verbal cues, creating a seamless and harmonious experience as they navigate different sex positions.

8. Addressing Challenges: Navigating Discomfort and Concerns

Challenges may arise during the exploration of sex positions, and this section provides guidance on addressing discomfort, concerns, or insecurities. Effective communication becomes a tool for navigating challenges, fostering a safe space for partners to express their needs and preferences.

9. Rituals of Intimacy: Creating Meaningful Moments

To conclude the exploration of sex positions, this section introduces the concept of rituals of intimacy. From creating a sensual ambiance to incorporating meaningful gestures, couples are encouraged to infuse their exploration with intentional moments that deepen their connection.

In the intricate tapestry of intimate relationships, the exploration of sex positions becomes a shared odyssey of pleasure, connection, and mutual discovery. By approaching this exploration with openness, communication, and a sense of adventure, couples can weave together a narrative of intimacy that transcends the physical act and becomes a celebration of their unique connection.

4.1 Intimacy as a Form of Communication

In the realm of intimate connections, the language of love often transcends verbal expression. This exploration delves into the profound concept of intimacy as a form of communication, unveiling the ways in which physical closeness, emotional attunement, and shared vulnerability become powerful avenues for expressing the depth of connection between partners.

1. *The Silent Dialogue: Communicating through Touch*

Intimacy, at its core, is a silent dialogue communicated through touch. This section unravels the significance of physical closeness, from tender caresses to passionate embraces, as a language that conveys affection, desire, and a profound understanding that goes beyond the limitations of spoken words.

2. *Emotional Resonance: Sharing the Unspoken*

Emotions, often elusive in verbal expression, find a home in the language of intimacy. This section explores how shared vulnerability, moments of tenderness, and unspoken understanding between partners create an emotional resonance that forms the foundation of a deep and meaningful connection.

3. Attunement to Non-Verbal Cues: The Dance of Connection

Partners engage in a dance of connection where non-verbal cues become the choreography. This section delves into the art of attunement, encouraging couples to be present and receptive to subtle gestures, glances, and body language that convey a wealth of emotions and desires.

4. Unveiling Desires: Passionate Expression

Intimacy provides a canvas for unveiling desires in a passionate symphony. This section explores how physical closeness becomes a conduit for expressing individual and shared desires, creating a space where partners feel free to communicate their most intimate longings without inhibition.

5. The Power of Presence: Being in the Moment

Presence becomes a potent communicator in the language of intimacy. This section emphasizes the transformative power of being fully present with a partner, creating a sacred space where the shared experience unfolds organically, fostering a profound connection in the present moment.

6. *Trust and Vulnerability: Building Bridges*

Intimacy serves as a bridge between trust and vulnerability. This section delves into the interplay of trust and vulnerability in the language of physical connection, highlighting how a safe and intimate space allows partners to express their deepest selves without fear of judgment or rejection.

7. *Intimacy Beyond the Bedroom: Everyday Expressions*

The language of intimacy extends beyond the confines of the bedroom. This section explores how everyday expressions of affection, such as a gentle touch, a knowing look, or a heartfelt gesture, weave a continuous thread of connection that sustains the intimate bond between partners.

8. *Shared Rhythms: Navigating Life's Challenges*

In times of joy and challenge, intimacy becomes a shared rhythm that couples navigate together. This section explores how the language of physical and emotional closeness becomes a source of strength, support, and solace as partners face the ebb and flow of life's myriad experiences.

9. *Rituals of Intimacy: Nurturing the Connection*

To conclude the exploration, this section introduces the concept of rituals of intimacy. From shared moments of relaxation to intentional acts of kindness, couples are encouraged to cultivate rituals that nurture the connection, reinforcing the language of intimacy as an ongoing and evolving expression of love.

In the intricate dance of relationships, intimacy emerges as a profound form of communication, speaking volumes without uttering a word. By embracing this language of love, partners embark on a journey of mutual understanding, shared vulnerability, and a connection that deepens with each tender and unspoken moment.

4.2 Finding Comfort and Connection

In the sanctuary of intimate relationships, the pursuit of comfort and connection forms the cornerstone of a fulfilling and enduring bond. This exploration delves into the art of finding solace in one another, fostering a deep sense of comfort, and weaving the threads of connection that withstand the tests of time.

1. *The Refuge of Emotional Comfort: Shared Warmth and Understanding*

Emotional comfort is the bedrock of connection. This section illuminates the sanctuary created by shared warmth and understanding, emphasizing the importance of being a source of solace for one another in moments of joy, sorrow, and everything in between.

2. *Vulnerability as a Bridge: Deepening Connection*

Vulnerability acts as a bridge to connection. This section explores the transformative power of sharing one's true self, fears, and aspirations.

By embracing vulnerability, partners cultivate an atmosphere where connection deepens, and the intimacy of being truly seen and accepted flourishes.

3. Creating Sacred Spaces: Nurturing Intimate Environments

The physical spaces we share become sacred grounds for connection. This section delves into the art of creating intimate environments—whether within the home or shared experiences—that invite comfort, fostering a sense of belonging and closeness between partners.

4. Shared Rituals: Building Foundations of Connection

Rituals, both big and small, become the building blocks of connection. This section explores the significance of shared rituals, from daily routines to special traditions, as mechanisms that reinforce the bond between partners and create a sense of continuity and stability.

5. Non-Verbal Resonance: The Language of Touch and Presence

Communication transcends words through the language of touch and presence. This section delves into the profound impact of non-verbal communication, encouraging partners to be attuned to the silent signals that convey love, reassurance, and a profound sense of connection.

6. Shared Laughter: The Joyful Thread of Connection

Laughter, a universal language, threads joy into the fabric of connection. This section explores the role of shared laughter in fostering connection, providing a lighthearted and essential counterbalance to life's challenges.

7. The Art of Listening: Cultivating Connection through Presence

Listening becomes an art that cultivates connection. This section emphasizes the transformative power of attentive listening, where partners offer each other the gift of being heard and understood, deepening the bonds of intimacy.

8. Connection Beyond Words: Intimate Silence and Understanding

Intimate silence becomes a language in itself. This section explores the moments of quiet understanding, where partners share a space of connection that transcends the need for words, cultivating a profound sense of unity and mutual comprehension.

9. Weathering Storms Together: Strength in Mutual Support

The storms of life become opportunities for connection. This section explores how partners, in supporting each other through challenges, strengthen the ties that bind them. Facing adversity together becomes a testament to the resilience of their shared connection.

In the tapestry of comfort and connection, couples embark on a journey of mutual support, understanding, and the creation of a shared sanctuary. By weaving these threads deliberately and with love, partners nurture a connection that not only withstands the trials of life but continues to flourish, deepening with each shared moment of solace and joy.

Chapter Five: Enhancing Bedroom Bonds

Within the intimate confines of the bedroom, the exploration of connection takes on a unique and passionate form. This chapter delves into the art of enhancing bedroom bonds, inviting couples to embark on a journey that transcends the physical, fostering a deep and meaningful intimacy that extends far beyond the realm of the sensual.

1. Setting the Scene: Creating an Intimate Atmosphere

The bedroom becomes a canvas for intimacy. This section explores the importance of setting the scene—creating an ambiance that invites connection and comfort. From lighting to decor, partners are encouraged to craft a space that enhances the sensual experience and fosters emotional closeness.

2. The Dance of Sensuality: Exploring Touch and Connection

Sensuality becomes a dance of connection. This section delves into the exploration of touch, caresses, and the art of physical connection. Partners are invited to embrace the language of sensuality as a means of deepening their bond and expressing desire in ways that transcend the ordinary.

3. Shared Fantasies: Nurturing Intimate Desires

Fantasies become a shared landscape for exploration. This section encourages partners to communicate and explore their intimate desires, creating a space where shared fantasies can be expressed without judgment. The open dialogue around fantasies fosters trust and deepens the connection between partners.

4. Mindful Presence: Being Fully Engaged in the Moment

The power of presence amplifies intimacy. This section explores the concept of mindful presence, encouraging partners to be fully engaged at the moment, free from distractions. By cultivating a sense of mindfulness, couples deepen their connection and elevate the shared experience to new emotional heights.

5. Communication Beyond Words: The Language of Desires

Desires find expression in the unspoken language of connection. This section explores how partners can communicate their desires beyond words, using non-verbal cues, body language, and shared energy to enhance intimacy. The subtleties of this communication deepen understanding and heighten the emotional resonance between partners.

6. *Exploring New Horizons: Introducing Variety and Creativity*

Variety becomes a catalyst for exploration. This section invites couples to explore new horizons in the bedroom, introducing variety and creativity to their intimate experiences. From trying new positions to incorporating different sensations, partners are encouraged to embrace the excitement of the unknown.

7. *Mutual Satisfaction: Focusing on Shared Pleasure*

Pleasure becomes a shared journey. This section emphasizes the importance of mutual satisfaction, encouraging partners to prioritize each other's pleasure and explore ways to enhance the overall experience. The focus on shared pleasure fosters a reciprocal and fulfilling connection.

8. *The Afterglow: Nurturing Connection Post-Intimacy*

The moments after intimacy become a time for connection. This section explores the importance of the afterglow—nurturing the emotional connection in the aftermath of physical intimacy. Partners are encouraged to engage in tender moments, fostering a sense of closeness and affirmation.

9. *Building Intimacy Beyond the Bedroom: Integrating Connection into Daily Life*

Bedroom bonds extend into daily life. This section emphasizes the integration of intimacy into everyday experiences, fostering a continuous connection between partners. From affectionate gestures to intentional moments of closeness, couples build a foundation of intimacy that extends far beyond the confines of the bedroom.

In the exploration of enhancing bedroom bonds, couples embark on a journey of profound connection, passion, and mutual discovery. By intentionally crafting a space for intimacy, communicating desires openly, and fostering a mindful presence, partners elevate their connection to new heights, creating a foundation of love and closeness that endures over time.

5.1 Introducing Variety

In the realm of intimate relationships, the introduction of variety becomes a dynamic force, breathing vitality and excitement into the shared experiences of partners. This exploration delves into the art of introducing variety, inviting couples to embark on a journey of discovery, growth, and the continuous evolution of their intimate connection.

1. *Embracing the Spice of Variety: Breaking the Routine*

Variety is the spice that infuses passion and vibrancy into intimate connections. This section encourages couples to break free from routine, embracing the excitement that comes with introducing variety. By stepping outside familiar patterns, partners open the door to new dimensions of intimacy and shared experiences.

2. Communication as a Catalyst: Expressing Desires and Boundaries

Effective communication becomes the catalyst for introducing variety. This section explores the importance of expressing desires and boundaries openly and honestly. Partners are encouraged to engage in a dialogue that fosters understanding, trust, and a shared vision for the exploration of new experiences.

3. Diverse Intimate Experiences: Expanding the Repertoire

Intimacy thrives on diversity. This section delves into the exploration of diverse intimate experiences, from trying new positions to incorporating different sensory elements. Partners are invited to expand their repertoire, cultivating an environment where creativity and variety enhance the depth of their connection.

4. Sensory Exploration: Engaging the Five Senses

Variety encompasses the engagement of all five senses. This section encourages couples to explore sensory experiences that extend beyond the physical, incorporating elements of touch, taste, smell, sight, and sound. By engaging the senses, partners create a multi-dimensional tapestry of intimacy.

5. Creating Intimate Adventures: Shared Exploration

Introducing variety becomes an adventure shared between partners. This section explores the concept of creating intimate adventures, whether through spontaneous moments of passion or planned explorations. The shared journey of discovery enhances the sense of connection and mutual excitement.

6. Novelty in Romance: Revitalizing Emotional Connection

Variety extends beyond the physical to revitalize emotional connection. This section delves into the role of novelty in romance, encouraging partners to infuse surprise, spontaneity, and thoughtful gestures into their relationship. Novel experiences become a source of rekindling passion and reinforcing emotional bonds.

7. Playfulness and Laughter: Lightening the Atmosphere

Variety is often accompanied by playfulness and laughter. This section explores the importance of lightening the atmosphere, and encouraging partners to approach new experiences with a sense of joy and humor. Playful interactions create a relaxed and open environment for exploration.

8. Shared Exploration of Fantasies: Mutual Respect and Consent

Fantasies become a terrain for shared exploration. This section emphasizes the significance of exploring fantasies with mutual respect and consent. Partners are encouraged to create a space where desires can be expressed openly, fostering a sense of trust and vulnerability in the shared exploration of intimate fantasies.

9. Adaptability and Flexibility: Navigating the Journey Together

Introducing variety requires adaptability and flexibility. This section explores the importance of being open to change and evolution in the intimate connection. Partners are invited to navigate the journey together, embracing the surprises and discoveries that come with introducing variety into their relationship.

In the rich tapestry of intimate connections, introducing variety becomes a transformative journey of shared exploration and growth. By cultivating a space for open communication, creativity, and mutual respect, couples embark on a path that enhances their intimacy, bringing excitement, novelty, and a continuous sense of discovery into the heart of their relationship.

5.2 Experimenting Safely

The path of intimate exploration is a dynamic journey where trust, communication, and mutual consent are the guiding stars. This exploration into experimenting safely invites couples to navigate the terrain of new experiences, ensuring a foundation of respect, consent, and emotional safety.

1. Establishing Open Communication: The Bedrock of Safety

Open communication serves as the bedrock for safe experimentation. This section emphasizes the importance of creating an environment where partners feel free to express their desires, boundaries, and concerns openly. Through transparent communication, couples lay the foundation for a safe and consensual exploration.

2. Mutual Consent: Respecting Boundaries and Desires

Mutual consent is the cornerstone of safe experimentation. This section delves into the concept of consent as an ongoing, enthusiastic agreement between partners. It explores how respecting each other's boundaries and desires fosters a sense of safety, ensuring that both individuals feel empowered and comfortable in the exploration process.

3. Setting Boundaries: Defining Comfort Zones

Setting clear boundaries becomes a proactive step in ensuring safety. This section encourages partners to define their comfort zones and communicate them to each other. By understanding and respecting these boundaries, couples create a space where experimentation can occur within the parameters of mutual agreement and emotional safety.

4. Establishing Safe Words: A Communication Lifeline

Safe words act as a communication lifeline during experimentation. This section explores the use of safe words as a tool for partners to communicate their comfort levels and immediately pause or stop an activity if needed. The establishment of safe words enhances trust and ensures that both individuals feel secure in their exploration.

5. Educating and Informing: Shared Awareness

Education is a key component of safe experimentation. This section highlights the importance of shared awareness about the activities and experiences being explored. Partners are encouraged to educate themselves, discuss their expectations, and approach experimentation with a mutual understanding of the potential physical and emotional aspects involved.

6. Prioritizing Emotional Safety: Nurturing Trust

Emotional safety is paramount in any exploration. This section explores how prioritizing emotional safety involves being attuned to each other's feelings, providing reassurance, and creating a non-judgmental space. By nurturing trust and emotional security, couples ensure that experimentation is a positive and enriching experience.

7. Checking In Continuous Communication during Exploration

Continuous communication is crucial throughout the process of experimentation. This section encourages partners to check in with each other regularly, assessing comfort levels and emotional states. Ongoing communication allows for adjustments, ensuring that the experience remains consensual and enjoyable for both individuals.

8. Embracing Gradual Progression: Building Comfort

Experimentation is a journey, and gradual progression is key to building comfort. This section explores the concept of taking small steps, allowing both partners to acclimate to new experiences at a pace that feels secure. Gradual progression enhances the sense of safety and builds trust in the exploration process.

9. Processing and Reflecting: Post-Experimentation Communication

Post-experimentation communication is as vital as the exploration itself. This section emphasizes the importance of processing and reflecting on the experiences together. Partners are encouraged to discuss their feelings, share feedback, and celebrate the positive aspects of the exploration, reinforcing a sense of connection and mutual understanding.

In the realm of intimate experimentation, prioritizing safety through open communication, mutual consent, and emotional security is the key to a positive and enriching journey. By navigating this terrain with respect, understanding, and continuous communication, couples cultivate a shared space where experimentation becomes a source of connection, growth, and profound intimacy.

Chapter Six: Overcoming Challenges

In the intricate tapestry of intimate relationships, challenges are inevitable yet navigable. This chapter explores the art of overcoming challenges, inviting couples to embrace resilience, open communication, and mutual support as they navigate the complexities that arise within the landscape of their shared connection.

1. Recognizing Common Challenges: Acknowledging Shared Realities

Understanding is the first step toward overcoming challenges. This section sheds light on common challenges faced by couples, such as communication breakdowns, differing expectations, and external stressors. By acknowledging these shared realities, partners gain insight into the complexities that can impact their relationship.

2. Communication Breakdowns: Bridging the Gap

Communication is both the challenge and the solution. This section delves into strategies for overcoming communication breakdowns, emphasizing the importance of active listening, empathy, and fostering an environment where both partners feel heard and understood. By bridging the communication gap, couples pave the way for effective problem-solving.

3. *Differing Expectations: Aligning Visions for the Future*

Differing expectations can create tension. This section explores the art of aligning visions for the future, encouraging couples to openly discuss their individual aspirations, values, and goals. By finding common ground and understanding each other's perspectives, partners foster a sense of unity and shared purpose.

4. *External Stressors: Navigating Life's Challenges Together*

Life's external stressors can test a relationship's resilience. This section provides insights into navigating challenges such as work-related stress, financial pressures, or family dynamics. By approaching external stressors as a team and supporting each other, couples build a foundation of strength and solidarity.

5. *Intimacy Concerns: Rekindling the Flame*

Intimacy concerns can be a delicate challenge. This section explores ways to rekindle the flame, fostering emotional and physical connection. From intentional gestures to seeking professional support, couples are encouraged to address intimacy concerns with compassion and a shared commitment to reigniting the spark.

6. *Trust Issues: Rebuilding and Strengthening Trust*

Trust is fragile but resilient. This section delves into strategies for rebuilding and strengthening trust when it has been compromised. By fostering transparency, demonstrating reliability, and engaging in open dialogue, partners can navigate the journey of rebuilding trust with patience and commitment.

7. *Balancing Independence and Togetherness: Harmonizing Individuality*

Balancing independence and togetherness is an ongoing dance. This section explores the importance of maintaining individuality within the relationship while nurturing a strong sense of togetherness. Partners are encouraged to support each other's personal growth and aspirations, fostering a dynamic equilibrium.

8. *Resolving Conflict: Turning Challenges into Opportunities*

Conflict is an inevitable part of relationships. This section reframes conflicts as opportunities for growth, providing tools for effective conflict resolution. By approaching disagreements with empathy, active listening, and a collaborative mindset, couples transform challenges into catalysts for deeper understanding and connection.

9. Seeking Professional Support: A Resource for Growth

Professional support can be a valuable resource. This section explores the option of seeking guidance from relationship experts, therapists, or counselors. By recognizing the value of external support, couples can navigate challenges with the assistance of professionals who provide tools and insights for growth.

In the journey of overcoming challenges, couples are invited to view difficulties as opportunities for strengthening their bond. By embracing resilience, fostering open communication, and supporting each other through the complexities of life, partners can cultivate a relationship that not only withstands challenges but thrives in the face of them, emerging stronger and more connected.

6.1 Addressing Common Concerns

In the intricate dance of intimate relationships, common concerns often arise, demanding thoughtful navigation and mutual understanding. This guide explores proactive approaches for addressing these concerns, providing couples with insights and strategies to strengthen their connection in the face of challenges.

1. Communication Breakdowns: Building Bridges of Understanding

Communication breakdowns are a common challenge. This section emphasizes the importance of building bridges of understanding through active listening, clear expression, and empathetic communication. By fostering an environment where both partners feel heard and valued, couples can address and overcome the hurdles of miscommunication.

2. Trust Issues: Rebuilding Foundations of Security

Trust forms the bedrock of strong relationships. This section delves into strategies for rebuilding trust when it wavers. Through open dialogue, transparency, and consistent actions that demonstrate reliability, couples can collaboratively rebuild the foundations of security and strengthen their bond.

3. Differing Expectations: Finding Common Ground

Differing expectations can lead to tension. This section explores the art of finding common ground by openly discussing individual aspirations, values, and goals. Partners are encouraged to align their visions for the future, fostering understanding and unity while embracing the unique qualities each brings to the relationship.

4. Intimacy Concerns: Cultivating Emotional and Physical Connection

Intimacy concerns are delicate but addressable. This section provides insights into cultivating emotional and physical connection. By fostering an environment of emotional openness, engaging in intentional gestures, and addressing concerns with sensitivity, couples can reignite the flame of intimacy and deepen their connection.

5. ***Balancing Independence and Togetherness: Fostering Harmonious Dynamics***

Balancing independence and togetherness is an ongoing process. This section explores the importance of supporting each other's individuality while nurturing a strong sense of togetherness. Partners are encouraged to communicate openly about their needs for space and closeness, fostering a harmonious and dynamic relationship.

6. ***External Stressors: Navigating Life's Challenges Together***

Life's external stressors can strain a relationship. This section provides insights into navigating challenges such as work-related stress, financial pressures, or family dynamics. By approaching external stressors as a united front and supporting each other through difficult times, couples build resilience and fortify their connection.

7. ***Resolving Conflict: Transforming Challenges into Growth Opportunities***

Conflict is an inherent part of relationships. This section reframes conflicts as opportunities for growth and understanding. By adopting effective conflict resolution strategies, such as active listening, compromise, and empathy, couples can transform challenges into catalysts for deeper connection and mutual growth.

8. Seeking Mutual Growth: Embracing Evolution Together

Individual growth is vital for a thriving relationship. This section explores the concept of seeking mutual growth, and encouraging partners to support each other's personal development. By embracing change together, couples navigate the evolving landscape of their relationship with understanding and shared enthusiasm.

9. Celebrating Successes: Fostering Positivity and Appreciation

Amid challenges, celebrating successes is crucial. This section highlights the importance of fostering positivity and appreciation within the relationship. By acknowledging and celebrating each other's achievements, both big and small, couples create a culture of mutual support and reinforcement.

In the journey of addressing common concerns, couples are empowered to navigate challenges with resilience, understanding, and a shared commitment to growth. By proactively addressing concerns and fostering a positive and collaborative environment, partners can fortify their connection, ensuring that their relationship not only endures but flourishes over time.

6.2 Seeking Professional Help

In the intricate landscape of intimate relationships, there are moments when seeking professional help can be a transformative and empowering choice. This guide explores the nuances of reaching out for professional support, offering insights and encouragement for couples navigating challenges that may benefit from the expertise of relationship professionals.

1. Recognizing the Value of Professional Support: Nurturing Relationship Growth

Recognizing the value of professional support is the first step. This section emphasizes the positive impact that seeking help can have on relationship growth. Whether facing communication barriers, trust issues, or other challenges, couples are encouraged to view professional assistance as a proactive step toward fostering a healthier and more resilient connection.

2. Identifying When to Seek Help: Signs and Considerations

Identifying when to seek help requires self-awareness. This section explores common signs that may indicate the need for professional support, such as persistent communication breakdowns, unresolved conflicts, or a sense of emotional distance. Couples are encouraged to consider seeking help when challenges surpass their ability to navigate them effectively.

3. Types of Relationship Professionals: Choosing the Right Support

Choosing the right type of support is essential. This section introduces various relationship professionals, including couples therapists, marriage counselors, and relationship coaches. Partners are guided to explore options that align with their specific needs and preferences, fostering a comfortable and effective environment for addressing challenges.

4. Taking the First Step: Initiating the Conversation

Taking the first step requires open communication. This section provides guidance on initiating the conversation about seeking professional help. Couples are encouraged to approach this dialogue with empathy, emphasizing the shared goal of strengthening their relationship and seeking support as a team.

5. Overcoming Stigma: Embracing the Path to Growth

Overcoming stigma is a crucial aspect of seeking professional help. This section addresses common misconceptions and encourages couples to view therapy or counseling as a positive and proactive choice. By embracing the path to growth, partners break down barriers and create a supportive space for their shared journey.

6. Setting Realistic Expectations: Understanding the Process

Setting realistic expectations is key to a positive experience. This section explores what couples can expect from the professional support process, including the collaborative nature of sessions, the timeframe for progress, and the role of active participation. Realistic expectations foster a mindset conducive to positive outcomes.

7. Confidentiality and Trust: Building a Safe Space

Confidentiality and trust are paramount in seeking professional help. This section emphasizes the importance of selecting professionals who prioritize confidentiality and creating a safe space for open communication. Couples are guided to foster trust in the therapeutic relationship, allowing for honest exploration and vulnerability.

8. Active Participation: Engaging in the Therapeutic Process

Active participation is the heart of therapeutic progress. This section encourages couples to actively engage in the therapeutic process, including open communication, self-reflection, and the implementation of strategies learned in sessions. Partners are empowered to take an active role in shaping the direction of their relationship journey.

9. *Integrating Learnings into Daily Life: Sustaining Positive Change*

Integrating learnings into daily life ensures sustained positive change. This section explores the importance of applying insights gained in therapy to real-life situations. Couples are encouraged to cultivate a mindset of continuous growth and apply the tools acquired during professional support sessions to enhance their relationship outside the therapeutic setting.

In the journey of seeking professional help, couples embark on a path of self-discovery, growth, and strengthened connection. By recognizing the value of support, addressing potential stigma, and actively participating in the therapeutic process, partners pave the way for transformative change and the creation of a resilient and thriving relationship.

Chapter Seven: Relationship Success through Intimacy

In the intricate dance of relationships, intimacy serves as the heartbeat that sustains the connection between partners. This chapter explores the profound significance of intimacy as the cornerstone for achieving relationship success. From emotional closeness to physical connection, the exploration of intimacy becomes a journey that weaves the threads of love, understanding, and enduring partnership.

1. The Essence of Emotional Intimacy: Building Deep Connections

At the core of relationship success lies emotional intimacy. This section delves into the essence of emotional connection, emphasizing the importance of vulnerability, shared experiences, and the mutual understanding that forms the foundation for enduring partnerships. Couples are invited to explore the depths of emotional intimacy, creating a space where true connection flourishes.

2. Nurturing Physical Intimacy: The Dance of Passion

Physical intimacy is a dance of passion that breathes life into relationships. This section explores the significance of physical closeness, from tender gestures to the exploration of desire. Couples are encouraged to nurture the flame of physical intimacy, recognizing it as a dynamic expression of love and a powerful force in building relationship success.

3. *Communication as the Bridge: Connecting Through Words and Actions*

Communication acts as the bridge that connects partners on multiple levels. This section highlights the role of effective communication in fostering intimacy, both verbally and non-verbally. By cultivating a language of love that includes open dialogue, active listening, and understanding, couples create a pathway to deeper connection and shared success.

4. *Rituals of Connection: Creating Meaningful Moments*

Rituals become the sacred threads that weave connection into the fabric of daily life. This section explores the significance of rituals of connection—whether through shared activities, heartfelt gestures, or intentional moments of togetherness. Couples are encouraged to infuse their relationship with meaningful rituals that strengthen their bond and contribute to long-term success.

5. *Trust as the Pillar: Fostering Security and Reliability*

Trust stands as the pillar that upholds relationship success. This section delves into the importance of trust in creating a sense of security and reliability. Partners are guided to understand the role of trust in fostering intimacy, where openness, honesty, and consistency become the building blocks for a resilient and successful connection.

6. Shared Dreams and Goals: Forging a Unified Path

Shared dreams and goals form a roadmap for a successful journey together. This section explores the significance of aligning aspirations and working towards common objectives. Couples are invited to envision their shared future, fostering a sense of unity and purpose that strengthens their bond and contributes to the success of their relationship.

7. Resilience in Adversity: Weathering the Storms Together

Resilience becomes the guiding force in facing challenges. This section examines how couples can navigate adversity hand in hand, relying on the strength of their connection. By embracing challenges as opportunities for growth and demonstrating resilience, partners fortify their relationship against the inevitable storms, ensuring its enduring success.

8. Continuous Growth: Evolving Together

Relationship success is an ever-evolving journey of growth. This section emphasizes the importance of continuous personal and relational development. Couples are encouraged to embrace change, support each other's individual growth, and evolve together as they navigate the dynamic landscape of their shared connection.

Celebrating milestones becomes a joyous affirmation of love and shared accomplishments. This section explores the importance of acknowledging and commemorating the milestones achieved along the relationship journey. By celebrating both small victories and significant milestones, couples create a culture of appreciation and reinforce their bond, contributing to the enduring success of their relationship.

In the tapestry of relationship success through intimacy, couples embark on a profound journey of connection, understanding, and shared growth. By nurturing emotional and physical intimacy, fostering effective communication, and embracing the challenges and joys of life together, partners create a resilient and thriving relationship that stands the test of time.

7.1 Building Lasting Bonds

In the intricate architecture of relationships, the art of building lasting bonds is a nuanced and deliberate process. This exploration delves into the foundational elements that contribute to the longevity and strength of connections between partners. From the cornerstone of trust to the intricate threads of communication, building lasting bonds becomes a purposeful endeavor that weaves a tapestry of love, resilience, and enduring commitment.

1. ***Trust as the Cornerstone: Foundations of Security and Reliability***

Trust stands as the unwavering cornerstone upon which lasting bonds are built. This section delves into the profound significance of trust in fostering a sense of security and reliability. Partners are guided to cultivate trust through openness, consistency, and mutual respect, establishing a foundation that withstands the tests of time.

2. ***Effective Communication: The Lifeline of Lasting Connections***

Communication serves as the lifeline that nourishes lasting connections. This section explores the art of effective communication, encompassing both verbal and non-verbal expressions. Couples are encouraged to foster a language of understanding, active listening, and empathy, creating a dynamic channel for the continuous exchange of thoughts, feelings, and desires.

3. ***Shared Values and Vision: Forging a Unified Path Forward***

Shared values and vision forge a unified path toward lasting bonds. This section examines the importance of aligning fundamental beliefs and goals. Partners are invited to explore and articulate their shared values, fostering a sense of unity and purpose that anchors their relationship amidst life's ebbs and flows.

4. Emotional Intimacy: The Heartbeat of Lasting Connections

Emotional intimacy forms the heartbeat that sustains lasting connections. This section delves into the depth of emotional closeness, emphasizing vulnerability, shared experiences, and the mutual understanding that deepens over time. Couples are encouraged to nurture the emotional bond that transcends the transient, creating a lasting and profound connection.

5. Adaptability and Resilience: Navigating the Journey Together

Adaptability and resilience become guiding virtues in navigating the journey of lasting bonds. This section explores how couples can embrace change, weather challenges, and grow together through life's inevitable twists. By fostering resilience and adaptability, partners ensure that their connection remains flexible, enduring, and capable of thriving in various seasons.

6. Rituals of Connection: Weaving Meaning into Daily Life

Rituals of connection weave meaning into the fabric of daily life. This section highlights the significance of shared activities, gestures, and intentional moments that become the threads binding partners together. Couples are encouraged to infuse their relationship with meaningful rituals, creating a tapestry of shared experiences that contribute to the lasting nature of their connection.

7. *Mutual Support and Empowerment: Building Each Other Up*

Mutual support and empowerment are the building blocks of lasting bonds. This section explores the transformative power of partners uplifting and empowering each other. By fostering an environment where both individuals feel supported in their personal growth and aspirations, couples create a lasting foundation of encouragement and strength.

8. *Celebration of Individuality: Nurturing Unique Identities*

The celebration of individuality nurtures the uniqueness of each partner. This section encourages couples to appreciate and honor each other's distinct identities, fostering a sense of autonomy and mutual respect. By valuing individuality, partners contribute to the lasting richness and diversity of their shared connection.

9. *Reflection and Gratitude: Sustaining the Essence of Connection*

Reflection and gratitude sustain the essence of lasting connection. This section emphasizes the importance of periodically reflecting on the journey together and expressing gratitude for the shared experiences. By cultivating a mindset of appreciation, couples contribute to the enduring vibrancy and depth of their lasting bonds.

In the artful construction of lasting bonds, couples embark on a deliberate and intentional journey. By weaving together trust, effective communication, shared values, and the threads of emotional intimacy, partners create a tapestry of connection that not only withstands the test of time but flourishes with every shared moment.

7.2 Sustaining a Fulfilling Relationship

The journey of sustaining a fulfilling relationship is a delicate dance, requiring intention, commitment, and continuous effort from both partners. This exploration delves into the art of nurturing a love that endures across time, encompassing the essential elements that contribute to a relationship's depth, resilience, and lasting fulfillment.

1. Cultivating Emotional Connection: The Heartbeat of Fulfillment

Cultivating emotional connection becomes the heartbeat that sustains fulfillment. This section delves into the depth of emotional intimacy, encouraging partners to prioritize vulnerability, understanding, and shared experiences. By nurturing the emotional bond, couples create a foundation that withstands the tests of time, fostering enduring fulfillment.

2. Prioritizing Quality Communication: The Bridge to Lasting Understanding

Quality communication serves as the bridge to lasting understanding. This section explores the importance of clear and empathetic communication, both verbal and non-verbal. Partners are encouraged to foster an open dialogue, active listening, and expressions of love that deepen their connection, ensuring sustained fulfillment in their shared journey.

3. *Shared Dreams and Aspirations: Fueling Mutual Growth*

Shared dreams and aspirations fuel the fire of mutual growth. This section examines the significance of aligning future visions and individual goals. Couples are invited to explore their aspirations together, fostering a sense of unity, purpose, and continuous growth that contributes to the lasting fulfillment of their shared journey.

4. *Acts of Love and Kindness: Nourishing the Relationship Daily*

Acts of love and kindness are the nourishment that sustains a relationship daily. This section emphasizes the importance of intentional gestures, supportive actions, and expressions of affection. Partners are encouraged to consistently show love in both grand and subtle ways, creating a tapestry of care that adds to the lasting fulfillment of their connection.

5. *Resilience in Adversity: Weathering Storms Together*

Resilience becomes a guiding force in weathering storms together. This section explores how couples can navigate challenges with strength and unity. By embracing adversity as an opportunity for growth, partners fortify their relationship against the inevitable storms of life, ensuring that fulfillment endures beyond moments of difficulty.

6. *Celebrating Milestones: Acknowledging Growth and Achievements*

Celebrating milestones becomes a joyful acknowledgment of growth and achievements. This section highlights the importance of commemorating shared successes, whether big or small. By recognizing and celebrating milestones, couples create a culture of appreciation that contributes to the lasting fulfillment of their shared experiences.

7. *Continuous Learning and Adaptation: Evolving Together*

Continuous learning and adaptation are vital in the journey of evolving together. This section encourages partners to embrace change, learn from experiences, and adapt to the evolving nature of their relationship. By fostering a mindset of curiosity and openness, couples ensure that their connection remains dynamic, fulfilling, and resilient across time.

8. *Individual Flourishing: Supporting Personal Growth*

Supporting individual flourishing enhances the richness of the relationship. This section explores the importance of allowing each partner to pursue personal growth and fulfillment. By supporting and encouraging each other's aspirations, couples contribute to a dynamic and flourishing connection that evolves alongside their individual journeys.

9. *Gratitude and Reflection: Savoring the Moments Together*

Gratitude and reflection are the savoring of moments that contribute to lasting fulfillment. This section emphasizes the significance of periodically reflecting on the journey together and expressing gratitude for the shared experiences. By cultivating a mindset of appreciation, couples contribute to the enduring vibrancy of their relationship.

In the pursuit of sustaining a fulfilling relationship, partners embark on a shared odyssey of love, growth, and mutual understanding. By prioritizing emotional connection, effective communication, and acts of love, couples create a relationship that not only endures but flourishes, ensuring lasting fulfillment in the tapestry of their shared life.

Conclusion

As we draw the curtains on our exploration of "Sex Positions: Understanding Sex Roles and Bedroom Bonds for Relationship Success," it becomes evident that the intricacies of intimacy extend far beyond the physical realm. This journey has transcended mere positions and techniques, delving into the profound interplay of emotions, communication, and the intricate dynamics that shape the intimate tapestry of relationships.

The essence of our exploration has been to illuminate the fact that the bedroom serves as a canvas for the expression of emotional connection, trust, and the mutual exploration of desires. Sex, in its myriad forms, becomes a powerful conduit for couples to deepen their bonds, foster understanding, and enhance overall relationship success.

Understanding sex roles has been a pivotal aspect of this journey, challenging traditional perspectives and inviting a more inclusive and communicative approach. It is not merely about the physical acts but about embracing the diversity of desires, preferences, and the unique dynamics that each individual brings to the intimate space. By acknowledging and respecting these differences, couples pave the way for a more harmonious and fulfilling connection.

Our exploration has also underscored the importance of communication in the bedroom. Open and honest dialogue about desires, boundaries, and fantasies lays the groundwork for a shared understanding that transcends the physical act. The bedroom becomes a space for vulnerability, trust, and the uninhibited expression of love, contributing significantly to the overall success of the relationship.

Moreover, the dynamics of desire and the introduction of variety have emerged as catalysts for relationship growth. Couples are encouraged to break free from routine, explore new experiences, and communicate openly about their fantasies. Variety becomes the spice that invigorates the connection, breathing life into the relationship and ensuring that passion remains a vibrant force.

As we conclude this journey, it is essential to recognize that the exploration of sex positions and intimate dynamics is not a one-size-fits-all endeavor. Each couple's journey is unique, and the key lies in embracing this uniqueness with an open heart and mind. It is about creating a space where partners feel safe to express themselves, where desires are heard, and where the intimate connection becomes a source of joy, fulfillment, and relationship success.

In the end, our exploration into sex positions has been a celebration of the multifaceted nature of intimacy. It is a celebration of love, trust, communication, and the ever-evolving dance between partners. May this understanding serve as a guide for couples on their journey towards lasting intimacy, deepening connections, and achieving relationship success in and out of the bedroom.